I0408402

Creating A Life of Consistency
AT YOUR OWN PACE

BY **LATRICE PACE**

Copyright © 2017 by Latrice Pace
All rights reserved. Except as permitted under the U.S. Copyright Act of 1976, no part of this publication may be reproduced, distributed, or transmitted in any form or by any means, or stored in a database or retrieval system, without the prior written permission of the publisher.

Bible references from the New American Standard Bible

ISBN-13: 9781544651897
ISBN-10: 1544651899

CreateSpace
Available from Amazon.com and other retail outlets
Available on Kindle and other devices

Written by Latrice Pace
Cover Design and Interior by Nations28/Kandice Phillips

DEDICATION

This book is dedicated to those who don't know what it means to give up.

INTRODUCTION

My name is Latrice Pace and I'm a creative being. I don't care to label myself as one thing because anything the creator put in me to do, I can do it. I'm also the author of an interactive self-help workbook entitled, Be the Change. However, many people know me as an entertainer, actress and singer. My most notable work was Nurse Nancy in Tyler Perry's production of *What's Done in the Dark*.

The motivation to make the necessary adjustments to my lifestyle came from frustration. I was simply frustrated with myself, my choices, my circumstances, my surroundings, MY LIFE. I was in desperate need for a change. I had experienced loss and was determined to not be the next casualty of something that I could control, if only I could get control. I lost my niece, my daddy, and my brother to illnesses that in my opinion could have been avoided by making consistent healthy lifestyle adjustments.

Consistently making the necessary lifestyle adjustments for a healthy existence were and are extremely challenging physically and emotionally. Physically, there were many times when my body would tell me that it had had enough, but I knew the truth. I had to surround myself with people and sometimes trainers that would push me beyond my mental limits, beyond my place of comfort. There were times I'd go walking and for the first 30 minutes it felt like someone was poking me with a million needles that had been set on fire. I knew that if I could manage to mentally block out the pain and discomfort, and endure the first 30 minutes that I'd be ok. After about a week of the burning needle syndrome, I was ok. It would never happen again, UNLESS I went a long period without working out again. It was only when I'd stop working out for a period, then start again.

The emotional adjustments were just as challenging as the physical ones were. I am such an emotional being. At the beginning of my journey, I probably cried every time I got on a treadmill, mainly because I didn't realize how I had been such a poor steward of my temple and secondly because of the burning needle syndrome. I gained control of my emotions through the Word of God. I saw my setbacks as opportunities to prove to myself that I could overcome anything that I might face. This was both my test and my chance and perseverance and resilience would be the catalyst to saving my own life. It is my deepest desire that my story and journey will not only inspire you, but also motivate you to fight to live. I hope you complete this book better equipped with the tools that you'll need to create the lifestyle you desire by making the necessary adjustments at your own pace.

I understand that we live in a society where people want the abbreviated answers to everything. Instant gratification has plagued our choices including the indulgence of things that would adversely affect our health and wellness. With that in mind, I started to name this *The Abbreviated Guide to Health and Nutrition*. I am also guilty. I don't mind reading, but I don't want to do a whole lot of reading. If I've finally found the motivation and inspiration to do a thing, I want the quick guide to get started and I only want 5 steps to get there.

In this book, I will give you a few steps to jump start your journey to health, healing and nutrition. As we grow together, I have included devotions for the mind, heart, body, and soul, strategically designed to keep you connected to the source that will fuel your life of consistency.

At the beginning of my health, fitness, and nutrition journey, there were things that I wished someone had told me that would have made my journey a little easier. I'm not sure if the information would have made sense to me at that time, but in hindsight I would have appreciated a heads up. The truth is that we all come to a point in our journey where no matter how much information we receive, it'll click when we are truly aligned and ready to receive insight and direction.

As an Integrative Health & Nutrition Coach I hope to show you where the light switch is, and empower you to flip it, but you will have to be willing to do the work to get up and flip the switch to ON. My purpose and intent is to create a path so clear to that light switch, that you will be compelled to get up and turn it on.

"Nothing happens until the pain of remaining the same outweighs the pain of change."- Arthur Burt

I am at the beginning of my Integrative Health & Nutrition Coaching career and I've already come to realize that change happens in many stages. Some people are just at the point where they've identified the need for change while others are more comfortable dissecting the process rather than taking action. Transforming your life takes a consistent commitment even when you don't feel like it. It is my goal to encourage each and every person that I reach to commit to change because you are worth it.

"If you're interested, you'll do what's convenient. If you're committed, you'll do whatever it takes."
- John Assara

WHERE DO I START?

Not only is this one of my most asked questions, it's also the question I asked myself when putting the ideas for this body of work together. I found it rather challenging to put together four short stepping stones to creating a life of consistency. There are so many components that play a key role in your success. However, I've managed to narrow it down for the sake of getting you started.

Let's start with the top four questions I'm asked all of the time. Where did you start? I've done many interviews where the interviewer wanted me to give their listeners a few quick tips as to where they could start. *Let's Go!*

This is just the beginning of a LIFELONG journey. I don't think people get that. This is for the rest of your life. Throughout our lives our goals change, our needs change, our desires and wants also change. To become successful at achieving any of these things, you must be patient and adopt an undeviating mentality.

Keep your eyes straight ahead; ignore all sideshow distractions. Watch your step, and the road will stretch out smooth before you. Look neither to the right nor left; leave (your old habits and mentality) in the dust.
Proverbs 4:26 MSG

START WITH BELIEVING

"Believe not only in God's ability to do for you, but believe in your ability to do, in Him, with Him, and through Him. If you do, you'll never be visionless. If you do, you'll have a limitless-boundless life, in this life and thereafter." -L. Pace, Certified Health &Nutrition Coach

1. Believe in yourself.
2. Renew your mind.
3. Believe in your ability to take control of your life.
4. Believe that small consistent changes will yield huge sustainable results.
5. No more self-criticism.
6. Surround yourself with people who will support your goals.
7. Practice daily devotions.
8. Set daily intentions so you will neither waste energy, time, nor become distracted.
9. Abandon your old story.
10. Stop rehearsing your old story.
11. Write a new story.
12. Make yourself a priority.
13. Be radical with self-care.
14. Think AND speak positively.

Forget about what's happened; don't keep going over old history.
Isaiah 43:19a

Be alert, be present. I'm about to blow your mind with something brand-new. Now it springs forth! It's bursting out! Don't you see it?"
Isaiah 43:19b

START WITH BELIEVING AND KNOWING THAT YOU ARE CAPABLE OF MORE.

While on my personal journey to health and wellness, I've learned that there are things that nourish us beyond what's edible. These things include both tangible and emotional things that can either add to our overall health or distract us from achieving our personal goals.

Relationships
Our relationships with our siblings, spouse, parents, co-workers, etc. should be intentionally nourished. We've all heard it before, "How we relate to others reflects how we relate to ourselves". If we are intentional about caring and nurturing ourselves, we will do the same for those we care about.

Career
It is important that you do what you love or find a way to enjoy the work you do until you can do what you love. Although many have done it and are now quite successful, it is not always realistic to quit your job to follow your passion. However, making adjustments to make your job an enjoyable "in the meantime" experience, is an expression of gratitude. The expression of gratitude does not suggest that everything is perfect, rather, it acknowledges the good and creates an internal dialogue that shifts our focus on provision, gratitude for connections, gratitude for the opportunity to experience growth and gratitude for grace.

A Strong Spiritual Practice
Be intentional about starting your day with prayer and meditation. Creating a devotional period can include breathing exercises, quoting a mantra or affirmation, declaring victory over situations, and/or reading or reciting a scripture. Your spiritual practice will keep you aligned and on track with what you believe. Let nothing compromise or come before you connecting with your source before you start your day. It is essential to setting the tone for your day.

Physical Activities
Experiment with a variety of activities until you find one that you truly enjoy. It is important that your physical activities don't feel like a chore or just another thing to scratch off your "to do" list. Your body was created to respond to movement, activities, and feeling productive. Movement stimulates you mentally, emotionally and spiritually. I think best when I'm at the gym. I come up with my best ideas when I'm on the stair master or just taking a stroll in the park and breathing in God. Be intentional about moving daily.

Mentality

Today could be the day you stop doing that self-destructive, that self-sabotaging thing you do. Simple, but not so simple, make the decision *daily* to reclaim and heal your body. How? Feed your mind lively thoughts and your body, live foods. When lovely, pure, positive, thought worthy, truthful thoughts go in, those same types of words will come out of your mouth, manifesting lovely, pure, positive, thought worthy, and truthful actions and results.

"Do not copy the behavior and patterns of this world, but be transformed by the renewing of your mind. Then you will be able to test and approve what God's good, pleasing, and perfect will is."
Romans 12:2

Nutrition

Water play a vital role in the human body and how much
you drink can affect your health. Too much water could result in mineral deficiency or imbalance and too little could be the cause of dehydration, fatigue, and even headaches. Just like nutrition is bio individual, so is your water intake. On average, men should ingest about 13 cups per day and women about 9 cups per day, depending on your diet, lifestyle, and individual needs. Personally, I try to ingest 11 cups per day and that's not including the water content in fresh fruit and green leafy vegetables.

Green Leafy Vegetables

It never fails, every time I eat green leafy vegetables I feel refreshed and renewed. I feel alive! Did you know that in Traditional Chinese Medicine the color green is related to the liver, emotional stability, and creativity? Did you also know that without enough vegetables in your diet, over 90% of bile goes back to your liver, then your blood, eventually damaging your arteries? Eat your vegetables in its natural state or as close to it as possible. Try not to kill them by overcooking them.

Supplements

Just like nutrition and water intake, vitamins and supplements are bio individual. You should consult your physician to understand what your body is deficient in. Personally, I try to eat foods that will give me my daily nutrients instead of taking supplements. However, sometimes it's challenging to meet my daily needs and for that purpose I use supplements. When I started my journey, I was experimenting with new foods. I wasn't sure which foods gave me the nutrients I needed. I wasn't even sure which nutrients I was possibly deficient in. There are many ways to find out what your body may need. The first way is obviously through blood work.

Another way is through electro dermal screening. I had a screening done and found out my deficiencies.

I have listed a few of the supplements that are now staples for me and more than likely what most of us are deficient in.

NECESSARY SUPPLEMENTS
- Multi-vitamin
- Fish oil (capsules or liquid. I like putting the liquid in my smoothies or over boiled eggs in the morning).
- Probiotic & Prebiotic for gut health. Another alternative is komucha (fermented teas, available at a health food store) or an apple cider vinegar tonic.

DETOX COCKTAIL
8oz of water
1 tsp of raw honey
1 TBSP Braggs apple cider vinegar (the brand I trust)

The beginning of any illness begins in the gut. Ever wondered why our parents and grandparents would always make us take cod-liver oil when we got sick? Gut Health! Their strategy was that a good cleaning would eliminate the bad bacteria and let the body heal itself with rest, proper nutrients and water.

Probiotics aid in digestion by cleaning out the gut so things can flow. Prebiotics feed your probiotics. I heard this story and it has stuck with me. Remember the arcade game Pac-Man, where the yellow Pac-Man eats his way through a maze of dots? Relating this to prebiotics and probiotics within your gut: Pac-Man is the probiotic and the dots are prebiotics.

PROBIOTIC
- Vitamin D (bone and teeth health) cardiovascular health, healthy immune system, brain and nervous system. Need I go on?

CREATE A REALITY THAT IS REAL

Our perceptions and beliefs tend to shape our reality, when TRUTH should shape our reality. Another's opinion of you is their view, it's not your truth. This not only relates to health and nutrition, but to our emotional and mental health as well.

How does the old adage go?
Sticks and stones may break my bones, but words will never hurt me.

Lies! It doesn't matter how tough our exterior persona may appear to be, what we've heard others say about us can become so ingrained in us that it will begin to distort the truth of who we really are. We must not process others opinions as facts.

You have no room for skepticism and doubt. You must be strategic in surrounding yourself with positive support that will dispel the opinions of others and help you create your new story based on truth. There was an exercise given to me in health and nutrition school to help me decipher what is an opinion versus facts.

FACT FINDER EXERCISE
A local newspaper reports that
"A 33-year-old man was arrested yesterday." - FACT
"The cop was courageous in his pursuit of the suspect." - OPINION

Throughout my journey, I often heard individuals voice their opinion that no matter how much weight I lost, that my butt and hips weren't going anywhere. So, it didn't matter how many squats, leg lifts, lunges or how long I stayed on the stair master, at some point their opinion became truth to me. It affected my effort and consistency. Why workout if my hips and butt aren't going anywhere? Nothing is going to change. I wasn't persuaded by either facts or opinion. It is truth and only truth that has freed my mind. We must combat facts and opinions with truth and the truth is, if I don't grow weary in doing good, If I continue to consistently workout, in due season I will reap the benefits, but only IF I DO NOT GIVE UP (Galatians 6:9 paraphrased).

Let me hold fast the confession of my hope for health, healing and wholeness without wavering, for He who promised to satisfy with long life and show his healing power is faithful (Hebrews 10:23; Psalm 91:16 paraphrased).

Now that you can distinguish between what is an opinion, fact, and truth, let's eliminate the limiting beliefs imposed on you by others that you have perceived to be truth. Let's establish what you believe about yourself. Belief is the beginning of health and healing. It is the beginning of a healthy self. It is the path to heal thy self.

What do you truly believe? If you need a little help I'll go first.

- I believe in myself
- I believe my goals are realistic.
- I believe that I will reach my goals.
- I believe that I am capable of making food choices that will help heal my body.
- I believe that I am loved and supported.
- I believe that a fulfilled physical activity will energize and motivate me.
- I believe that what I think will influence my actions.
- I believe that small adjustments will yield sustainable results.

CREATING A LIFE OF CONSISTENCY

It has happened to all of us. We will get this burst of inspiration to start a new workout regimen or dietary theory, then two weeks later we have either plateaued, swearing it off as non-effective or become bored and ready to switch it up. Even if you fall off the wagon, dust yourself off and get back in there. Mistakes are proof that you are trying. You are doing your best and tomorrow you will do better.

In my experience, the key to consistency is simply being intentional about EVERYTHING you do. We are all familiar with the saying, "fail to plan, plan to fail". IT'S TRUE! Everything around you responds to clarity, so set an intention. Your intention is your compass. It will keep you from wasting energy. Declare EXACTLY what you want. Are your daily activities moving you closer to or farther away from your goals?

No more wasted energy! One of the main things that set me on the wrong path was being misguided by a spiritual leader I trusted for guidance. I realized that I had spent years accomplishing his goals and supporting his vision without setting any of my own. If you don't set goals for yourself, you are doomed to achieve the goals of someone else. There's nothing wrong with supporting someone else's vision, but in some way, it should be aligned with the vision and goals you have set for yourself. In my opinion you should benefit in some way. It can be benefits of provision to accomplish your goals. It can be information or knowledge, "the how-to" to accomplish your goals. It can be connecting you with people to help you accomplish your goal. I don't feel that your motive should be to personally gain, but in some way, you should gain.

BE INTENTIONAL ABOUT PREPARING

Every Sunday night I take a few moments to prepare myself for another week of working out and making healthy food choices, maybe even meal prep. I prefer to meal prep if it's not a travel week. I tell myself, THIS IS WHAT WE ARE GOING TO DO! I prepare my mind. I prepare my food. I prepare my workout clothes by making sure they are all clean AND DRY. There have been times I'd wash and forget to place them in the dryer and if it's already a challenge for you to get up and do some sort of physical activity, all you need is for something like that to happen to make it more challenging and even cause you to change your mind.

BE INTENTIONAL ABOUT PLANNING

If you're interested you'll do what is convenient, but when you're committed you will do whatever it takes.

There was so much I didn't know, but Google makes everybody an expert. I would Google everything and go with what resonated with me. There is a lot of misinformation out there, but I tried it all until I found that thing that spoke to me. It's all trial and error. You must be willing to experiment. Don't use not knowing or not having help as an excuse, do whatever it takes to educate yourself. Do whatever it takes to win by planning to win. Plan your meals. I know that life happens fast and schedules are busy, but make processed foods and fast food an absolute last resort.

To Effectively Plan:
Release, Realign, and Reconnect to God's purpose, will and intent.

Readjust and Refine
Eliminate anything and anybody who is not beneficial to the journey nor the destination.

Redefine
If you're not making headway with a goal,

Recalibrate and Release
Move on towards something that is more aligned with your core values. Give yourself permission to let go of the old goals and be more deliberate with the new ones.

Be honest with yourself. Set deadlines and reminders. Notice and target specific areas of distraction that may cause you to procrastinate. Develop an anchored strategy that is realistic.

BE INTENTIONALLY PERSISTENT

You will not always feel like working out, but do it anyway. You will not always feel like making the healthier choice, but find a compromise and do it anyway. You will not "eat clean" (see guide to eating clean) all the time, but eat as clean as possible, when you can, where you are, and per your budget, don't sweat it.

You will fall off the wagon, but when you do, redefine your activities and choices. Perhaps you tried to accomplish too much too soon. Remember gradual changes will be most effective. Perhaps you set some unrealistic goals in your past attempts. Create support so you won't get lonely. There is strength in numbers. Workout with friends who are also serious about their health and wellness.

"A person standing alone can be attacked and defeated, but two can stand back-to-back and conquer. Three are even better, for a triple-braided cord is not easily broken." Ephesians 4:12 NL

BE INTENTIONAL ABOUT PARTING

You must be willing to part with old habits, negative people, and doubting mentalities. Let go of stagnant people. It doesn't mean you don't love or care for them, you just love and care for yourself more. Let go of stagnant generational patterns. The sins and decisions of the generations before you are not your destiny.

BE INTENTIONAL WITH PRAISING YOURSELF

Cut yourself some slack. You should celebrate your accomplishments. If you are completely goal driven and never take moments to celebrate and praise yourself or you don't allow others to praise you, you will eventually become burnt out, bored, uninspired and unmotivated.

SUCCESS TO ME

When you define success and your goals, you will eliminate counterproductive activities. Define what success in this area of your life looks and feels like so that once you're there, you'll be aware. Then you can go on to set other goals. Once you define what success looks like to you, you won't become discontented while reaching your goals. You won't become discontented once you reach your goal, and most importantly, you will not be tempted to compare your personal accomplishments with another.

DEFINE IT

Success to me looks like:

_____
_____
_____
_____
_____
_____
_____
_____
_____
_____
_____

Success to me feels like:

_____
_____
_____
_____
_____
_____
_____
_____
_____
_____

Trust the process. It's not going to happen overnight. When you're interested, you will do what is convenient. When you're committed, you will do whatever it takes. BE committed, BE the change!

CLEAN EATING

"Eating clean is about being empowered with knowledge, making the best choices that we can, going easy on ourselves, and doing the best that we can do from day to day. - Terry Walters

BASIC Principles
- Keep it whole
- Get in the kitchen, cook, and prepare your own meals
- Eliminate refined sugar and carbohydrates
- Maintain a healthy blood sugar
- Remember the magic combination of protein, fat, and a complex carbohydrate.

DEVOTE THEN DEVOUR

I have been able to be consistent on this journey because daily I recommit my allegiance, fidelity, and faithfulness to this never-ending journey.

Daily devotion connects you to self and to having a strong spiritual core. Just like our health and nutrition, our spiritual practices are bio individual. The examples below are how I maintain my spiritual practice. We can't embark upon a life of consistency without knowing how to connect to our source, our center.

- Prayer
- Devotion
- Peaceful Meditation

WHY PRAY?
Prayer aligns your will and thoughts with God's. And don't forget your armor, your shield and weapon from every weapon.

Put on the whole armor of God, that ye may be able to stand against the wiles of the devil. Ephesians 6:11 KJV

Prayer turns insults into humor. It helps you to focus in the face of distractions. You will find inspiration when discouragement is riding your back. You are strengthened for every task and attack ahead. You can't afford not to start your day with prayer.

PRAYER FOR CONSISTENCY

Father, I thank you for strengthening me to complete this workout. I release my mind and body of any unrealistic expectations from a single workout. Today, my food choices will assist in healing and not hurting my body. My food choices will be aligned with your purpose, your will and intent for my temple.

Knowing the results of these two consistent acts of faith will in time be evident. Tonight, I will sleep in gratitude and I will rise with thanksgiving in my heart, prepared and ready to do it all again tomorrow.

DEVOTION ONE

WAIT PATIENTLY
Remember, "it's a marathon, not a sprint"!

I've always been a go getter. Once I conceive of an idea and have prepared my mind to get it done, I am already on the track and at the 100-meter mark. Forget the starting line, save the, "on your mark, get ready, set, go", I'm gone! Many times, I'd make it to the finish line with no injuries and feeling like a champ. Other times I felt the effects of not warming up before hitting the track.

Waiting is preparation. When I began writing new music for my live recording, waiting was one of the most difficult things to do. The first day I pulled away to write I was so excited that I started having meetings, planning dates, and comparing tape truck estimates. One morning God gently said, "I told you to write, perfect the songs I have given you. I didn't tell you to set any dates." LOL!

What would happen if farmers became impatient with harvesting their crop? Releasing kingdom music that has not been perfected is like trying to get someone to enjoy fruit out of season. You know what it should taste like. It's kinda good, but something is missing. It's not ripe, sweet, nor savory. It's not ready.

The blessing in waiting is taking advantage of the opportunity to be prepared and perfected. The first thing I'd ask myself when I kept getting anxious to set a date, share or announce something was, "WHY?" Waiting reveals your motives and the moment you make a seemingly small move with the wrong motives, it shifts you out of an assisted race into a solo race. Waiting strengthens your dependency on God.

I am so in the place where I'm not doing ANYTHING without his approval. I didn't set out to record this year, HE DID! So, this is his gig, not mine.

Waiting refines you. This process is purifying me and has removed unwanted elements from my mentality, ideas, and even how I deal with and see people.

In closing, remember that in your waiting, there is a purpose and you aren't waiting alone. God is very strategic and mindful of you. He's after a desired result that only comes from going "the long way". He's after a desired result that is perfected in private along the journey so that it is not exposed in public at the destination.

WAIT PATIENTLY - READING
"But they who wait for the Lord shall renew their strength; they shall mount up with wings like eagles; they shall run and not be weary, they shall walk and not faint…" - Isaiah 40:31

WAIT PATIENTLY - INTENTION
Just wait, patiently. No anxiety. Throughout the day ask yourself, "why?" Check in with your motives.

WAIT PATIENTLY - PRAYER
Our father in heaven, hallowed be your name, your kingdom come, your will be done, on earth as it is in heaven. Today I will wait for the Lord. I will be strong and have hope in his word. I will not envy others who are prospering. My hope is in you Lord. I thank you that every need is met, every divine connection is made, and all hindrances and distractions are no more. Forgive me of my debts as I forgive my debtors. And lead me not into temptation, but deliver me from the evil one, deliver me from unproductive thoughts, and deliver me from negativity, even in my mentality. For thine is the kingdom, and the power, and the glory, forever. Amen.

DEVOTION TWO

PEACE AND QUIET GOODNESS

I love learning from Native Americans and Indians all over the world. In my opinion, they have such a reverence for God, nature and His creation. I became captivated when studying their beliefs about cross species transference. The character traits of the animal you ate can be transferred to humans and you essentially become more like the species you eat. Wow, right?!

Indians are just that in sync with the earth, one with nature and I'm simply fascinated by their history, language, and culture. For instance, The Kekchi Indians of Guatemala, define peace as quiet goodness, which is close to the meaning of the Hebrew word Shalom. I absolutely love this definition, quiet goodness! It conveys the idea of something that is active and aggressive, not the absence of disturbance.

The biblical concept of peace is to be complete, whole and to live well. It has nothing to do with what's going on around you, but everything to do with what's going on inside of you. I paraphrased Philippians 4:7-8, the peace of God which is beyond human understanding, shall guard your heart from stress and worry, and guard your mind from things that aren't lovely, pure, just, virtuous, and praiseworthy.

How to obtain quiet goodness?
Be at peace with God. You can be at peace with God by receiving his gift, Christ. Christ brings peace. I see it as one of the many gifts that comes with accepting him. When we receive Jesus Christ, we cease being enemies of God and we are now at peace with God.

"Peace I leave with you; my peace I give you. I do not give to you as the world gives. Do not let your hearts be troubled and do not be afraid." John 14:27 NIV

I NEVER saw this until reading a commentary one day. In John 14:27. Jesus said, "my peace I give you." He gave us something that personally belonged to him. He gave us his peace that kept him in "quiet goodness" when he was betrayed, abandoned, rejected, carried the sins of the world, falsely accused, mocked, abused, stabbed, wounded, and killed. He said look, at some point in life you're going to be faced with one if not several of these at once. Don't be afraid and don't worry because the same quiet goodness I had, now belongs to you. You can face it, go through it and you will come out alright and un-phased by external situations.

PEACE AND QUIET GOODNESS - READING
"Now may the Lord of peace himself give you peace at all times and in every way. The Lord be with all of you." 2 Thessalonians 3:16

PEACE AND QUIET GOODNESS - INTENTION
I intentionally want to be in fellowship with God. I intentionally receive Christ and grab hold to all of the gifts he has made available. I intentionally will be in quiet goodness today regardless of any external situations.

PEACE AND QUIET GOODNESS - PRAYER
Our father in heaven, hallowed be your name, your kingdom come, your will be done, on earth as it is in heaven. Forgive me of my debts as I have forgiven my debtors. Father, I receive your peace on today, your quiet goodness. Lead me not into temptation, but deliver me from the evil one: For thine is the kingdom, and the power, and the glory, forever. Amen.

DEVOTION THREE

A RESTORED SOUL

While reading Psalms 23: 1-3 it became clear to me that God is into luxury spa treatments. It is so apparent! The Lord is my shepherd I shall not want. THAT'S LUXURY! I'M A KEPT WOMAN, LOL.

He maketh me to lie down in green pastures. He continues to place me in situations where I have to trust him for my daily bread, for my provision.

He leads me beside the still waters. SPA! RELAXATION! REST! When I read this I immediately visualized myself walking out of a noisy existence into the spa where everything is suddenly quiet, calm and relaxing. The ambience is filled with melodic harp and water instrumentals. Still waters, that is part of the stream where no water currently is visible, that place where there is no gravity. Nothing and no one is pulling at your energy.

He restoreth my soul: he leads me in the paths of righteousness for his name's sake. SPA! He continually restores me, He replenishes me and returns me to my natural state. He makes me normal again, lol. Not just the me people see, but the essence of who I am, my soul.

So how are we continually restored? Go back to verse 1. Stop striving and grinding. Acknowledge he is the good shepherd and you have no want. Lie down in his provision. Follow him beside the still waters and be restored. Ladies, it's like being out with your man. Although you may have your own resources, you know you don't have to use them because you're with your man. Noooo, I am not about to say Jesus is my man! Being in the presence of our significant other makes us feel safe, cared for, provided for. We have no want. That's how it is in the presence of the Lord.

A RESTORED SOUL - READING
"And after you have suffered a little while, the God of all grace, who has called you to his eternal glory in Christ, will himself restore, confirm, strengthen, and establish you." 1 Peter 5:10

A RESTORED SOUL - INTENTION
To not want. To be content with today's bread/provision. Walk beside still waters. Let nothing or no one pull at your energy. Walk the path of righteousness and be restored.

A RESTORED SOUL - PRAYER

Our father in heaven, hallowed be your name, your kingdom come, your will be done, on earth as it is in heaven. Today I thank you that every need is met, every divine connection is made, and all hindrances and distractions are no more. Forgive me of my debts as I have forgiven my debtors. And lead me not into temptation, but deliver me from the evil one: For thine is the kingdom, and the power, and the glory, forever. Amen

DEVOTION FOUR

POWER & STRENGTH

For God has not given us the spirit of fear, self-doubt, and no confidence; but he has given us the ability to produce an effect, the ability to influence others, physical might, mental strength, love, and a sound mind that has been revived, rescued, and reserved for His thoughts.

In addition to power, he has also given us strength, the ability to do things quickly. I love making physical fitness and spiritual parallels that are life applicable. In physical fitness, strength is the ability to move a certain amount of weight, whereas power is the ability to move weight quickly.

Immediately Matthew 17:20 comes to mind. "…if you have faith as small as a mustard seed, you can say to this mountain, 'Move from here to there,' and it will move."

Our faith is our power and strength and activating it makes nothing impossible. We can "do" and "do quickly."

We don't even have to exert our physical strength to get results. All we have to do is *speak.*

POWER & STRENGTH - READING
"May you be strengthened with all power, according to his glorious might, for all endurance and patience with joy." Colossians 1:11

"I can do all things through Christ who strengthens me." There's a version I love that says,

"….through Christ who infuses me with his supernatural ability."
Philippians 4:13

POWER & STRENGTH - INTENTION
Believe God's Word. Acknowledge fear(s). Activate God's Word. Dismantle fear(s) by bringing every thought and every lie into the obedience of Christ, His Word. Meditate on today's reading.

POWER & STRENGTH - PRAYER
Our father in heaven, hallowed be your name, your kingdom come, your will be done, on earth as it is in heaven. Today I walk in boldness, strength, courage, confidence, and power. I thank you that every need is met, every

divine connection is made, and all hindrances and distractions are no more. Forgive me of my debts as I have forgiven my debtors. And lead me not into temptation, but deliver me from the evil one: For thine is the kingdom, and the power, and the glory, forever. Amen

DEVOTION FIVE

SELF VALIDATION

If I had to name one thing I didn't like, it would have to be waiting on someone else for anything. I can't do it. It's relinquishing control of my time to someone who more than likely will not value it. Yeah, I can't do it. I'd rather make my own plans, fill you in and you can feel free to join me if you like.

It's interesting how we can be so strong and mature in one area, but like a little kid in another. When it comes to my creative expressions, I often find myself wrestling with the inner kindergartener who runs to her daddy for validation after completing her coloring activity.

Do you like it?
Will you tell all of your friends?
Will you frame it and put it on the wall?
Will you, will you, will you?

As an adult, I've come to realize that I've always wanted my daddy's validation, but never got it. I can't blame him. I'm the ninth child, the eighth daughter. By the time he got to me he was probably all out of affirmations. However, the very last thing he said to me before he made his earthly transition, as he looked at me with surprise was, "Girl, you are more powerful than you know."

That one sentence made up for every moment I wanted his approval and acceptance, and never got it. God often gives me really cool ideas. I found myself running the ideas by people I thought were important to me, those whose opinions I valued. They would never respond as if they never received my email or text.

One day God checked me. He made me aware that my asking people what they thought about what he had given me was low key seeking their validation, approval, and acceptance, and not trusting him. I wasn't ok with God's approval of me. His acceptance wasn't enough.

Seeking validation is our way of wanting to be accepted. One of the most alarming lessons I'm currently learning is that you can work with, hang out with, laugh with, create with, spend time with some people, and they will never accept you. Not being accepted is a disheartening distraction, but the moment YOU DECIDE to show up for yourself, be present for yourself, validate and accept your thoughts, ideas, and feelings, that is the moment you will become more powerful than you know.

SELF VALIDATION - READING

"Open up before God, keep nothing back; he'll do whatever needs to be done: He'll validate your life in the clear light of day   and stamp you with approval at high noon." Psalm 37: 5-6 MSG

SELF VALIDATION - INTENTION

Pray. Do not seek approval, acceptance or validation from man, not even in the smallest, most subtle or seemingly harmless way. Show up for self. Be present for self. Validate self. Accept self. Trust God, he validates and approves.

SELF VALIDATION - PRAYER

Our father in heaven, hallowed be your name, your kingdom come, your will be done, on earth as it is in heaven. Today I thank you that every need is met, every divine connection is made, and all hindrances and distractions are no more. Forgive me of my debts as I have forgiven my debtors. And lead me not into temptation, but deliver me from the evil one: For thine is the kingdom, and the power, and the glory, forever. Amen

DEVOTION SIX

INHALE EXHALE

Breathing is the only function that allows you to change the function of the nervous system. Improper breathing is the root of many health problems especially in the digestive system. Do you realize that as you breathe, the breath of God fills your lungs and when done properly, promotes healing within your body?

INHALE EXHALE - READING
"The Spirit of the Lord has made me; the breath of the Almighty gives me life." Job 33:4

"The LORD God formed the man from the dust of the ground and breathed into his nostrils the breath of life, and the man became a living being." Genesis 2:7

INHALE EXHALE - INTENTION
Control your emotional state by breathing. Before responding or reacting, take a moment and breathe. When feeling stressed or when your body tenses up, *breathe*. Breathe deeply, slowly, quietly, and frequently, while sitting down.

INHALE EXHALE - PRAYER
Our father in heaven, hallowed be your name, your kingdom come, your will be done, on earth as it is in heaven. Today I ask for wisdom, wisdom to know when I'm taking on more than you intended. Lord show me how to set boundaries, boundaries that honor you and my temple. Help me not to shut down that which I don't understand. Today I will be open to new ways of managing stress and maintaining inner peace. Lord, breathe the breath of life into me today. I thank you that every need is met, every divine connection is made, I am aligned, and all hindrances and distractions are no more. Forgive me of my debts as I have forgiven my debtors. And lead me not into temptation, but deliver me from the evil one: For thine is the kingdom, and the power, and the glory, forever. Amen

DEVOTION SEVEN

FULFILLMENT

Many of us spend days, weeks, months, years, even decades busying ourselves with activities that aren't fulfilling. When was the last time you did something for someone else and it left you with a feeling of utter satisfaction and happiness? It's the best feeling in the world.

The awesome thing about fulfillment is that once you experience that "my life has meaning" feeling, you're never satisfied with that one occurrence. You'll want it to be at the end of everything you do. Fulfillment is a journey that requires connecting with, trusting in, and total reliance on God.

Fulfillment's seed is sown in the silence and watered with peace. It is that inner knowing that all you do is God orchestrated and for His glory. Fulfillment grows in the sunrays of thankfulness and gratitude, allowing us to be present in every moment, releasing us from anxiety, discontentment, inner conflict, and increasing our well-being.

FULFILLMENT - READING

You make known to me the path of life; in your presence there is fullness of joy; at your right hand are pleasures forevermore. Psalm 16:11

FULFILLMENT - INTENTION

If you notice all of the previous words and phrases are interrelated and connected. You can't obtain one without the other. Today's intent is to reflect, create some quiet time, pray, meditate, breathe deeply, be at peace, be open to creative expression, to be in the moment and free of anxiety, to live in a place of gratitude and express your thankfulness by first being kind to yourself and then others.

FULFILLMENT - PRAYER

Our father in heaven, hallowed be your name, your kingdom come, your will be done, on earth as it is in heaven. Today I'm asking and believing that you will make my life's path known. I thank you that I will find fulfillment and overwhelming joy in your presence today. Father, I thank you that every need is met, every divine connection is made, every hindrance and distractions are no more. Forgive me of my debts as I have forgiven my debtors. And lead me not into temptation, but deliver me from the evil one: For thine is the kingdom, and the power, and the glory, forever. Amen

DEVOTION EIGHT

SELF DOUBT

Self-doubt is something I'm sure all of us can write about, from the most successful to the yet striving. If you think about its core definition, it's one of the most hurtful things we can do to ourselves. Imagine loving and knowing someone all of your life, then one day an ugly truth is revealed, they don't trust you and think you are unreliable. That would crush me to the core. I would immediately want to know what have I done to cause such distrust. Well that is essentially what self-doubt is. It's telling yourself that your thoughts, ideas, and motives can't be trusted. It's like looking yourself in the mirror and saying, "you're unreliable" AND YOU BELIEVE IT!

Foolishly, I threw my confidence away at a very young age. I got caught in the comparison trap early on. I thought I could never measure up to my older siblings so I just didn't try. Let me save myself the time and effort because I'll never be able to do it like that one. I laugh about it now because I no longer doubt myself. God has restored my confidence. When trying to overcome anything it's important to have a strong spiritual practice and read the Word of God. It's your tool, your weapon to overcome. It was with the Word of God that I was able to banish self-doubt and gain self-confidence. It'll pop its head up every now and then, but the Word of God is the burden of proof to every lie we are presented with.

I can take you through EIGHT STEPS TO SELF CONFIDENCE, but let's just get to the core of it, chop its ugly head off with our sword, THE WORD, THE TRUTH, AN UNDERSTANDING OF WHO GOD CREATED YOU TO BE.

SELF DOUBT - READING
"In the love of the Lord there is strong confidence." Proverbs 14:26

"So we can confidently say, "The Lord is my helper; I will not fear; what can man do to me?" Hebrews 13:6
"Have I not commanded you? Be strong and courageous. Do not be frightened, and do not be dismayed, for the Lord your God is with you wherever you go." Joshua 1:9

"Let no corrupting talk come out of your mouths, but only such as is good for building up, as fits the occasion, that it may give grace to those who hear." Ephesians 4:29

"The Lord will fulfill his purpose for me; your steadfast love, O Lord, endures forever. Do not forsake the work of your hands." Psalm 138:8

SELF DOUBT - INTENTION
I will think well of myself. I will speak well of myself. My posture will be of confidence and boldness. I will sever all ties with any associations that do not strengthen and build me up.

SELF DOUBT - PRAYER
Father, help me to see myself the way that you see me. Teach me to love myself the way that you love me. Show me how to wear my crown of confidence and boldness, Amen.

DEVOTION NINE

ANXIETY

We've talked about trust and analyzed just how reliant we are or in some cases not reliant on God. If we continue to push ourselves beyond our physical limits for more money, position, or even fame we aren't trusting Him to do much. A dysfunctional focus on those things will lead to stress and stress has become an epidemic today.

Ironically today I wanted to talk about ANXIETY and believe it or not, anxiety is a reaction to stressful situations. We become stressed because according to us, God either isn't moving at all, he isn't moving fast enough, or he isn't moving the way we want him to.

If you see the picture I'm painting, it all goes back to yesterday's word, TRUST. We can't trust God because we don't trust ourselves or anyone else. We've proudly adapted this me, myself, and I mantra and we are happy on our islands alone. I know because I'm talking about myself. You have ONE time to let me down or not come through for me, especially after I've built up enough courage to finally admit that I need you or need help. I guess I should say, that's the old me. I'm intentionally trusting myself and others, but ultimately trusting God when I make the decision to trust others.

When it comes to trust, you should ask yourself, "what am I afraid of?" Whatever happened is in the past, IT HAS HAPPENED. Do not be a prisoner to history. Do not spend another moment of your right now or tomorrow trying to prevent what happened yesterday. That makes no sense. It happened, it hurt, you lived through it, you've learned, and as you heal, you will learn to attach the RIGHT emotions to that experience so you're not anxious and living in fear of it happening again.

ANXIETY - READING
"Give your entire attention to what God is doing right now, and don't get worked up about what may or may not happen tomorrow. God will help you deal with whatever hard things come up when the time comes." Matthew 6:34 MSG

ANXIETY - INTENTION
I intend not to worry. I intend not to stress, not dwell on the past and not think about tomorrow. I intend to live in today, to increase my physical and

mental energy by practicing your deep breathing for 10 minutes. I will simply deep inhale and long and controlled exhales.

ANXIETY - PRAYER

Our father in heaven, hallowed be your name, your kingdom come, your will be done, on earth as it is in heaven. Father, teach me how to trust you. I don't want to be a prisoner of my past. I don't want to worry about tomorrow. I want to be present in what you are doing in and around me today. I don't want to forfeit my peace so I throw every care and concern at your feet.

Today I thank you that every need is met, every divine connection is made, and all hindrances and distractions are no more. Forgive me of my debts as I have forgiven my debtors. And lead me not into temptation, but deliver me from the evil one: For thine is the kingdom, and the power, and the glory, forever. Amen

DEVOTION TEN

MEDITATION

Meditation is Philippians 4:8 in action, turning your mind to a single point of reference. Whatever things are lovely, pure, just, virtuous, praiseworthy, think on these things. Meditation reduces stress, improves concentration, and my favorite is that it increases self-awareness.

MEDITATION - READING
But his delight is in the law of the LORD, And in His law he meditates day and night. Psalms 1:2

On the glorious splendor of Your majesty And on Your wonderful works, I will meditate. Psalms 145:5

MEDITATION - INTENTION
Today's intention is to keep your attention away from distracting thoughts and focus on the present moment. To I will enter a state of rest and relaxation to achieve inner peace.

MEDITATION - PRAYER
Our father in heaven, hallowed be your name, your kingdom come, your will be done, on earth as it is in heaven. Help me to access perfect peace on today as I meditate and keep my mind on you. Lead me by still waters and restore my soul. Today I thank you that every need is met, every divine connection is made, and all hindrances and distractions are no more. Forgive me of my debts as I have forgiven my debtors. And lead me not into temptation, but deliver me from the evil one: For thine is the kingdom, and the power, and the glory, forever. "My meditation of Him shall be sweet: I will be glad in the LORD." (Psalms 104:34) Amen

DEVOTION ELEVEN

GRATITUDE

Gratitude is taking the time to notice and reflect on the things you are thankful for. Many healing-holistic counselors will suggest keeping a gratitude journal and logging what you are grateful for at the end of your day. Honestly, I have about five incomplete journals. I'll see a really pretty one, buy it and promise to be faithful to it. I'll go hard for about two weeks and, oh well. The practice isn't about a perfect logging record, but doing it as much as you remember to do it and doing it ESPECIALLY when you're feeling discontented.

Gratitude is a state of being that realigns and shifts your focus. Gratitude can significantly increase your well-being and your overall life satisfaction. Gratitude will cast a countenance of compassion and kindness on you that is easily transferable to your surroundings.

GRATITUDE - READING
Rejoice always, pray continually, give thanks in all circumstances; for this is God's will for you in Christ Jesus. 1 Thessalonians 5:16-18 NIV

Rejoice always...Be cheerful no matter what -MSG; Be glad-hearted - AMP.

GRATITUDE - INTENTION
Today and forevermore, devote yourself to maintaining a state of gratitude. You have no complaints, *NOT ONE.*

GRATITUDE - PRAYER
Our father in heaven, hallowed be your name, your kingdom come, your will be done, on earth as it is in heaven. Help me to establish and maintain a state of gratitude, knowing that it aligns and shifts my focus to your will. Your will is for me to give thanks in and for all things. Today I thank you that every need is met, every divine connection is made, and all hindrances and distractions are no more. Forgive me of my debts as I have forgiven my debtors. And lead me not into temptation, but deliver me from the evil one: For thine is the kingdom, and the power, and the glory, forever. Amen

YOUR NEW DAILY PRACTICE

BREATHE

LEAVE WORK ENERGY AT WORK

CONTROL YOUR ATMOSPHERE, IT'S YOUR SACRED SPACE

DISCONNECT, RECHARGE, RECONNECT, REPEAT

CLOSING THOUGHTS

"Your body will change, people will walk away,
life will happen!

You have to make it your mission to continue to find and recreate "that thing" that keeps you going, that physical activity that and keeps you mentally healthy.' And doesn't cause harm to neither you nor others.
-Latrice Pace

ABOUT THE AUTHOR

LATRICE PACE

Born into Atlanta's First Family of Gospel, Latrice was destined to venture into the ministry of music. Having nine siblings to precede her, all artist in the Gospel Industry, she felt it was necessary to create a path of her own. Latrice discovered her passion for acting and began to travel with various live theatrical productions and shows which she enjoys very much.

"I was born into the business; and to be honest, I wanted nothing to do with music. I felt everybody in the family was already doing it so I needed to do something different. However, my daddy made sure I knew that Gospel music was a family ministry and there was no such thing as "doing something different". Once I graduated from high school I began to sing in the group with my sisters. Shortly thereafter I began to travel with my oldest sister, Shun, as her assistant/road manager. I believe serving her for years opened so many other doors to work with various artist as well as the arts.

I've been in the music industry for 20 years and in the arts (Urban Theater) for about 15 years. I learned early on that I was my own walking/traveling business. So, with my experience along with the influence of my mentor Donald Lawrence, I'm learning that it's not just about having a professional image before people, but it's important that every aspect of you, your life, your business – be legitimate and professional. I also have future aspirations to mount my own theatrical production, but during this chapter of my life, L. Pace Entertainment, LLC is about being smart in this business of music. I don't want to do what I do out of necessity, but simply because I love to do it.

WHAT'S HAPPENING NOW?
Visit my website for exciting Health & Nutrition Coaching offers. www.latricepace.com

Visit my social media outlets for updates
Twitter: iamlatricepace
Facebook: Latrice Pace
Linkedin: Latrice Pace
Instagram: theatricalpace

Visit my blog for recipes
latrcepace.wordpress.com

WHAT'S NEXT?
Live recording of original inspirational music, March 27, 2017. Visit the website for updates and details. www.latricepace.com

www.ingramcontent.com/pod-product-compliance
Lightning Source LLC
Chambersburg PA
CBHW071308280526
45788CB00004B/1857